MW01167130

Women, Assertiveness, and Health

A rationale for the use of assertiveness training in promoting women's health

DECEMBER 1990

A report produced for the Health Education Authority

Research undertaken and report compiled by

Lesley Pattenson MSc, DHSA, DipHEd
Co-ordinator of Women's Health Education,
Health Education Authority

and

Jan Burns MSc, PhD, C. Psychol. AFBPsS
Lecturer in Clinical Psychology, University of Leeds/
Yorkshire Regional Health Authority

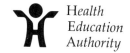

Health
Education
Authority

© Health Education Authority 1990
Hamilton House
Mabledon Place
London WC1H 9TX

ISBN 1 85448 174 6

Typeset by BookEns Limited, Baldock, Herts.
Printed in England by Belmont Press

Contents

Summary

• By reviewing relevant literature, this paper explores and clarifies the links between women's health and assertiveness and related concepts, in order to legitimise assertiveness training (AT) as an effective and appropriate technique for use by those concerned with women's health education and health promotion.

• Assertiveness is a way of communicating clearly, effectively, and without anxiety, based on respect for self and others. There is a close correlation between high levels of assertiveness and high levels of self-esteem, self-confidence, self-concept, self-efficacy, internal locus of control, self-actualisation, and self-empowerment.

• There is a close correlation between a lack of assertiveness and anxiety, depression, low levels of the attributes referred to above, and general physical and mental symptomatology.

• Women tend to be less assertive than men because of the socialisation process into the passive 'feminine' roles, and because of the circumstances of most women's lives. Women also tend to suffer more from mental health problems and have generally lower levels of self-confidence than men. Levels of assertiveness are also related to, and affected by other factors, including race, ability, age, sexuality, and social class.

• There are many areas in which assertiveness, or a lack of it, is related directly to decision-making with regard to health behaviours, such as smoking, drinking, use of contraception, and so on. Failure to carry out decisions often lies in the inability to communicate effectively with others, which in turn is closely related to assertiveness skills.

• AT is effective in promoting change, both in terms of specific behaviours and overall self-esteem, self-confidence, health, and well-being, and in generally improving health. AT can lead to improvements in many aspects of women's lives, such as drug use, relationships, sexual health, anxiety, menopause, participation in health care, and so on.

• Women have redefined and extended the limits of what are traditionally considered to be women's health issues to include not only the prevention of ill-health, but the promotion of a better quality of life through access to information and through greater choice and control over their health, bodies, and lives. The contribution AT can make to enabling the attainment of greater choice and control is clear.

• AT, which originated as a method of psychological treatment for patients, is now widely used by women as a self-help measure to learn how to improve communication and to develop self-esteem and self-confidence, as well as to deal more effectively with difficult interpersonal situations.

• AT can enhance the effectiveness of all approaches to health education. It can be tailored to suit different levels and models of health education, and is a particularly powerful technique in the enhancement of self-empowerment, which should be at the root of all approaches to health promotion. The parallels with life-skills teaching are clear: life- and social-skills training are widely accepted and used in school health education, but the potential of similar work with adult women in the community has not yet been adequately recognised by health educators.

• Women's access to AT, and approaches which make clear links with AT and health should be acknowledged as central to the work of all those concerned with promoting women's health. Appropriate resources which clarify and build on these links are needed. The particular needs of specific groups should be targetted by offering AT, taking full account of differences in social and cultural context. (An HEA project is currently developing such resources. Details are given in Appendix A.)

Preface

This paper was commissioned by the Health Education Authority (HEA) as part of a programme of work exploring and developing the links between assertiveness training (AT) and women's health education. It is of relevance to all health educators – whether theorists, policy-makers, or practitioners – who have any remit or interest in skills training and/or promoting women's health.

By identifying and clarifying the interrelationship between health, health-related behaviour, and assertiveness and associated concepts, we aim to provide a rationale for the development of AT techniques and programmes as a valid tool for use by a variety of people involved with health education, particularly those working with women. We also aim to promote a clearer understanding of assertiveness not simply as a type of interaction between two people, but as a whole way of life based on high self-esteem, respect for self and others, and increased control over one's life and decision-making, in addition to improved social and communication skills.

We will present research findings which link assertiveness, or a lack of it, with different aspects of health or health behaviours; and also draw parallels between the principles and practice of AT and the various theoretical and practical approaches to health education, health promotion, and disease preventive health care. In this way we aim to legitimise the use of AT within the health field, and dispel any misunderstandings and misgivings which may have arisen from its recent popularisation among women.

While the focus of this paper is on the relevance to women's health, AT could also benefit men's health, and we do not wish to minimise its value in men's health education. Women in particular, however, have a heritage of being positioned socially, psychologically, and politically as the dominated group, and therefore have an impetus to assert themselves. This is reflected in the fact that it is women who have been quick to realise the relevance of AT to their lives, while on the whole men have not yet recognised its potential.

The Health Education Authority is concerned mainly with the primary prevention of ill health through promoting individual behaviour change. This paper therefore focuses on aspects of personal health, and does not explore the relationship of assertiveness to community health issues, or the potential use of AT in facilitating change for the wider population.

Notes on the literature reviewed

The remit of this research was to review the existing academic and research literature in order to provide a scientific framework demonstrating the links between assertiveness and women's health. The review did not on the whole consider the many books which are now available on assertiveness through the popular press. (For a bibliography, see Whitehead, 1990.) Consequently the available academic literature imposed a number of constraints which should be acknowledged:

1) The roots of assertion and AT lie firmly in psychological theory and practice, originating from an individualistic and treatment-orientated approach aimed at psychopathological individuals. In contrast, most of the AT now undertaken, and the sort that is of relevance to health educators and those working in the community, is undertaken in a group context, and not aimed specifically at individuals who are considered ill, or who have a psychological disorder. Frequently it is chosen by people seeking a self-help method outside the traditional healthcare system. Whitehead (1990) notes that many women 'use assertiveness as a vehicle within their work in order to encourage women to build their confidence and self-esteem'.

2) Because much AT is done outside the professional sphere, evaluation of its effectiveness is done for the benefit of the trainer for the improvement of future course presentation, rather than for submission to the academic or professional journals. Consequently there is a skew in the available research literature which overrepresents the type of AT used as a therapeutic tool by professionals, and fails to identify and assess the sort of AT which women in the community have developed, and are sharing with others as a means of learning personal skills and promoting general self-development.

3) Much of the original psychology data was gathered from the most accessible populations, that is, patients and (often psychology) college students. Generalisations made from such atypical populations should be regarded cautiously as there is evidence to show that levels of assertiveness are influenced by many variables, including sex, race, culture, class, and personal value systems – as well as the socio-political climate within which the subjects live. However, there is a dearth of literature that focuses in any depth on the relationship between these factors and assertiveness.

4) Most of the literature is North American, and has to be viewed in the context of social, cultural, and political differences between the United States and Britain, as well as differences in health education and health care policies and delivery.

5) Probably because the links between assertiveness and health are largely implicit and complex, there is little research that has focused specifically on the relationship between women's health and assertiveness, or AT.

6) Even where evaluations of the benefits of AT in treating, preventing or promoting some health condition or behaviour have been done, it must be remembered that there is no such thing as a standard AT course in terms of aims and objectives, or course content and methods. This is not, however, a disadvantage since flexibility is vital in meeting the specific needs or circumstances of the group of participants.

Notwithstanding these constraints, we believe we present ample evidence linking assertiveness with women's health and supporting Furnham's (1979) view that:

Behaviour modificationists, social skills trainers, and popular writers agree on two basic beliefs with regard to assertiveness: (1) lack of assertiveness is a major cause of feeling of unease, anxiety and inadequacy; and (2) assertiveness is the product of a set of learned attitudes that can be changed, unlearned, or relearned.

Introduction

Historical perspective

Assertiveness training is not new. The concept was originated by psychologists working on behaviour therapy
and social skills in the United States in the 1940s and
1950s (Salter, 1949; Wolpe, 1958). However, AT has tran-
scended its position as 'one of the fundamental therapeutic interventions of the behaviour therapist' (Galassi
and Galassi, 1978) used to treat 'pathological' behaviours
in their patients, to become an educational method
widely used to promote both specific skills and general
well-being among the 'well' population.

AT has had an increasingly popular following in Great
Britain since the mid-1970s, when, noting the success of
classes in the United States, Anne Dickson was instru-
mental in promoting the development of courses in this
country (Dickson, 1982). Since then AT classes have flour-
ished in various forms throughout the country and
within various organisations, run by a variety of trainers
including, for example, health education officers, community workers, speech therapists, tutors in further education establishments, youth workers and those involved
in the voluntary sector (Whitehead, 1990).

AT has been used widely by women returning to
employment, as well as in other areas of life, and the
majority of participants continue to be women. The reasons
for this are developed later in this book. It is important to
note that elements of AT have been subsumed under
various titles, such as management training, personal
effectiveness, confidence building, and so on.

What is assertiveness?

A variety of definitions of assertiveness, or assertive behaviour, have been postulated, evolving from the early behavioural ones to those encompassing central principles such as rights, responsibilities, and self-concepts. For example, Alberti (1974) suggests that assertiveness is 'Behaviour which enables a person to act in his own best interest, stand up for himself without undue anxiety, to express his rights without destroying the rights of others'. Here the term 'rights' refers to the assertion of the individual's rights to express their own thoughts and feelings.

Basically, assertiveness is a way of communicating clearly and effectively, particularly in difficult personal, social, and professional situations. Elements of assertive behaviour learned through AT include: making clear, specific requests; being able to say 'no'; giving and receiving criticism; managing the expression of feelings, especially anger; receiving compliments; taking the initiative; understanding nonverbal messages; building self-esteem; and improving self-presentation.

The distinction between assertion and aggression may sometimes be blurred. Indeed, some of the early behavioural tests included elements of aggression as a measure of assertiveness. Furthermore assertion in women is more likely to be interpreted as aggression. As there is a greater social disapproval of aggression in women than in men, Garrison and O'Jenkins (1986) suggest that assertive women may be generally less well liked, even when appropriately assertive, than are assertive men. Del Greco (1980) states that 'Assertive individuals learn to stand up for their rights without violating the rights of others. Assertive behaviour does not humiliate, threaten, dominate, degrade, or use coercion or threat.' The underlying principles of aggressive behaviour and assertive behaviour differ radically since assertive behaviour is based on respect for the other person, and aggression is not. Del Greco (1986) adds that generally the assertive person is considered confident, friendly, honest, respectful, caring, and aware of their own and others' feelings.

While AT can be of value to all people, whether they tend to behave passively, aggressively, or manipulatively, it must be remembered that the assertive person may choose not to behave assertively if they consider this inappropriate.

How is assertiveness related to health?

A conceptual framework of assertion and its relationship to health behaviour and the promotion of health is now presented. This framework is only one example from a number that could be used, and is presented to highlight how integral assertiveness is to health.

In terms of Maslow's hierarchy of needs – ranging from basic physical to self-actualisation – a variety of emotions is experienced that originate from the drive to fulfil these needs (Maslow, 1970), for example anxiety, which results when specific needs are not met. Such emotions and needs influence a person's decision-making processes, including those decisions that concern health behaviour. For example, decisions may be made concerning preventive health care, or reactive decisions may be necessary in response to specific health disorders. The resulting behaviour will affect the person's general state of health, which in turn will affect their hierarchy of needs, thus setting up a reinforcing system comprising a number of elements which can be affected by the presence or absence of assertiveness.

Tones (1986) illustrates the position of assertiveness within decision-making behaviour in the form of a model:

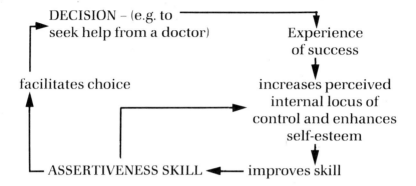

Figure 1 Assertiveness and decision-making
(Tones, 1986)

There is a huge number and range of areas in which assertiveness or a lack of it, is related to the outcome of health decision-making, for a decision is worthless if the person does not have the confidence and skills to carry out the required action.

Very often the barriers to carrying out such decisions lie in the person's inability to communicate effectively, for example the failure to refuse drugs, drink, or cigarettes when offered by someone persuasive; the failure to convince health professionals to provide certain health tests, or not to administer undesired treatments; the failure to negotiate safe sex or to end an abusive or destructive relationship; the failure to insist on healthy food choices in shops or catering establishments; the failure to influence improvements in health and safety in working practices or environments, and so on. Furthermore, repeated failure will lead to a lowering of self-confidence and self-esteem, resulting in additional negative effects on mental health.

There is clearly considerable potential in encouraging health-promoting choices by enabling the individual to communicate assertively in such situations, and this is well within the remit of those involved in health education, since, in a review of health education approaches, Kolbe *et al.* (1981) conclude that 'The appropriate functions of most health education programmes are both: a) to increase the competencies of individuals to make decisions about health related behaviours, and b) to increase those skills and inclinations required to engage in health conducive behaviours.'

Assertiveness and health education theory and practice

A holistic approach to health education – the importance of mental health

The oft-quoted 1946 World Health Organisation (WHO) definition of health as 'a state of complete physical, mental and social well being, not merely the absence of disease' although idealistic, was valuable because of its positive approach to the promotion of health and well-being, and also in drawing out the mental and social dimensions of health, in addition to physical health. By recognising their interdependence, it challenged health educators to adopt a more holistic approach towards health, while determining more realistic and achievable goals than those of the WHO.

Yet nearly half a century after the 1946 WHO definition was formulated, the measurement of health, both of individuals and communities, still tends to rest on epidemiological criteria of mortality and morbidity statistics (Barnes, 1987), and there is still considerable pressure on health educators to concentrate on modifying those aspects of health behaviour for which there is clear evidence of a resultant increased risk of mortality.

Inevitably, aspects of mental and social health are given low priority, and the promotion of mental health as a key objective is rarely found in practice. This is despite considerable evidence of the psychosomatic element of health and the recognition that improved mental health often leads to a reduction in physical symptoms. However, AT offers a 'multi-purpose' approach to health education in that it helps to develop competence in decision-making as related to physical health, and, in the longer term, increased assertiveness also enhances self-esteem and self-confidence, and reduces anxiety and other aspects of mental ill-health. Furthermore, AT improves social health through enhanced interpersonal relationships, due to the improvement of communication skills and the building of respect for self and others.

The relationship of assertiveness to different approaches to health education

A variety of approaches to health education has been described and schematised. One analysis is that of Tones (1986), who encapsulated them into the preventive, educational, and radical approaches, and argued that the goal of self-empowerment should underpin them all. The key components of self-empowerment are a perceived internal locus of control, and high self-esteem.

The *raison d'être* of the self-empowerment approach is to foster informed decision-making and action, hence 'improving health by developing people's ability to understand and control their health status to whatever extent is possible within their environmental circumstances' (French and Adams, 1986). In contrast, the preventive approach seeks to foster only healthy, disease-reducing decisions, as defined by the health educator, which, as already illustrated, still requires the skills to put such decisions into operation. Nevertheless, Tones suggests that self-empowerment could lead to a 'prudent' life-style rather than one that is health-damaging, since a self-empowered person may be better able to resist pressures to smoke, use alcohol or other substances, etc.

Anderson (1986) agrees that self-empowerment is central to health promotion, and argues that if health promotion is to succeed, self-empowerment is essential:

> For example, if publicity campaigns are to make an impact, their recipients need the self-esteem and skills to follow them up – the confidence to join a sports club, the assertiveness to ask people not to smoke, and, above all, the belief that they can have some influence over their health status.

Self-empowerment strategies seek to facilitate decision-making by modifying the person's self-concept and by enhancing self-esteem. This is achieved by equipping people with a variety of life-skills which not only modify their self-image, but also prove useful in their own right for attaining specific goals. Again, assertiveness figures as a key skill in this model, as illustrated by Tones (1986):

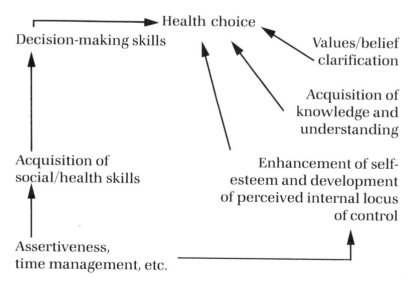

Figure 2 A self-empowerment approach to health education. (Tones, 1986)

The Life Skills Schools Health Education Programme materials (Hopson and Scally, 1979) are a direct application of the self-empowerment approach (Judge, 1985). Anderson (1986) identifies the five elements of self-empowered behaviour on which the programme is broadly based: awareness, goals, values, information, and life skills. These life skills include many of those learned through AT – being positive about oneself, relating to others, managing negative emotions, effective communication, managing conflict, and asserting oneself generally.

In fact, there are many similarities and links between AT and approaches already favoured or used by health educators, primarily with children and young people, such as personal and social education, life-skills training, and so on. The value placed on such approaches was clearly illustrated by a recent survey commissioned by the HEA (Anon, 1990), which assessed the current practices, development, and organisation of health education in schools. From 1,742 responses, it was noted that 41% of primary and 71% of secondary schools included assertiveness within their overall health education programmes, and work on self-esteem was included in 68% and 86% respectively.

It seems paradoxical that while assertiveness is being widely and routinely taught to children and young people within health education programmes, it is not yet as widely recognised and used by health educators working in adult health. Nevertheless, Whitehead (1990) found that 39% of 68 health education/promotion units surveyed provided some AT for women. Indeed the development of materials and approaches making specific links between assertiveness and health would provide health educators with an effective technique, since it is possible to vary the emphasis and structure of any AT programme to fit the goals of the health educator designing the course. Whatever the primary objectives of the health educator in using AT techniques, however, if internalised and put into practice effectively, assertiveness skills and techniques usually will lead to a gain in self-confidence, self-esteem, and self-control. Such a longer-term outcome is a bonus of the technique, and has longer-term, positive implications for the health of the person developing the skills.

Because AT operates on different levels, it is possible to conceptualise its relationship to the different approaches to health education/promotion. French and Adams (1986) place the various approaches in a heirarchy, in which they argue that methods that aim to change people's behaviour are of less value than those which aim to increase self-empowerment, the ultimate level being that of collective action, through which social and economic circumstances that affect health can be influenced. The relationship between assertiveness and these first and second levels has already been illustrated, and will be developed further in this paper. It must also be obvious that assertive individuals will be well placed to work for wider change alongside other members of the community.

Whichever approach to health education is preferred, at a theoretical or operational level, AT techniques have a positive contribution to make, and therefore are relevant to anyone concerned with preventive health care, health education, and health promotion. Whitehead (1990) suggests that:

> It would be useful to begin looking at assertiveness and women's health education as a process; one part of which may be about enabling women to gain more effective access to information and health care through developing their confidence and self-esteem. Another is perhaps about working with women to actually prevent and/or deal with potentially health threatening thought and behaviour patterns . . . it is a dynamic and preventative way of working which takes into account the perspective and contexts in

which people are needing to change. It draws on women's own experiences and values and encourages women to grow by validating those experiences. This is fundamental to learning theory and we should celebrate assertiveness for its simplicity, common sense and relevance to our whole being.

Part One
Assertiveness theory

Assertion as a 'clinical' concept and AT as 'treatment' have a long history, and are central to much psychological research and theories of psychological functioning. That assertiveness is bound to gender roles is also well justified from this research, which is expanded upon later. This next section positions assertion within the framework of psychological theory and research. It also draws links with other health-related concepts, and describes the aims and efficacy of AT.

Theories of assertion

There is a great deal of literature about assertiveness and AT, and it encompasses many different theoretical and methodological orientations. The many definitions of assertive behaviour reflect this variety. The early origins of assertion theory arose from the behaviourist school of Salter (1949) and Wolpe (1958). Wolpe developed a psychological model based upon a conceptual neurological framework, and explained assertion in terms of anxiety being ameliorated through 'reciprocal inhibition', i.e. trying to elicit a response contradictory to anxiety, such as assertive behaviour in a situation that usually provokes anxiety.

From a psychoanalytic point of view assertion is associated with the development of the super-ego. Put simply, a person possesses a certain amount of psychic energy that may be used in a variety of ways, including self-recrimination and coping strategies for distress (Freud, 1933). A certain degree of super-ego development is desirable and normal, but when this develops into an over-inhibition of self-expression and outgoing behaviour, AT is appropriate.

Dollard and Miller (1950) developed these ideas further in terms of learning theory. Like Freud they viewed inhibitions as deriving from early socialisation experiences, but explained them in terms of classical conditioning rather than through psychodynamic mediators such as the super-ego. In later life, situations arise that are similar to those in which the person experienced punishment in early life, and this creates anxiety. Anxiety is seen as an acquired drive, which the person attempts to reduce by behaving in certain ways, usually by escaping and not confronting. Unassertive escape responses do not allow the person to acclimatise to the fear-evoking circumstances, nor do they necessarily reduce the likelihood of the circumstances occurring again, so anxiety is always a response in these situations.

Rogers (1951, 1963), taking a more humanistic and client-centred approach based on Maslow's ideas of self-actualisation, postulated that people have a drive to reach their ultimate potential. Early experiences of inadequacy and unworthiness restrict and inhibit self-expression in order to avoid the anxiety and distress of not living up to one's full potential. It is not until the person experiences acceptance and nonjudgemental, positive regard that they are able to assert themselves and behave in a way that is congruent with their previously thwarted potential.

From such wide theoretical foundations, other definitions of assertiveness have arisen that incorporate elements of all these different models. For example, assertiveness is a behaviour that is 'positive, direct, courteous and goal orientated' (Bakker and Bakker-Rabdau, 1973; Phelps and Austin, 1987). It is also a behaviour that 'maximises the reinforcement value of social interaction'

(Heimberg *et al.*, 1977), and has been defined by Alberti and Emmons (1987) as 'enabling people to stand up for themselves without undue anxiety'. It seems reasonable that this type of behaviour should have a high social value, and this is indeed supported by research findings. For example, Kelley *et al.* (1983) note that this type of communication is likely to allow self-expression, ease conflicts, and elicit similar positive behaviour from others in conflicted intimate behaviour.

Additionally, Galassi (1973) and MacDonald (1975) note that unassertive behaviour may result from a failure to discriminate when assertive responses are necessary through a lack of assertive skills, or from a lack of knowledge about what constitutes an appropriate response. This is not in conflict with the developmental models of assertion, as one of the implications is that appropriate role models were lacking in early life. The ideas of Galassi and Galassi (1978) highlight the skills aspect of assertiveness, which has been adopted in social-skills training, where the acquisition of assertion skills is a fundamental part of any package.

Thus, although the major theorists have differing views about the ways in which unassertive behaviour can become habitual, they agree that inhibitive, unassertive behaviour originates from the person's experience during the developmental process (Rathus, 1975). They also agree that the motivation behind unassertive behaviour is the reduction of anxiety (Furnham, 1979). Nevertheless, the differing approaches and definitions make the task of measuring such a concept as assertiveness a complex task.

Measuring assertion

By far the most frequently used measures of assertiveness are the paper-and-pencil questionnaires that the subjects complete, often referred to as 'self-report measures'. Before 1970 there were few useful methods specifically used to measure assertiveness; interestingly, measures of anxiety or personality were used as tests of assertiveness (Galassi and Galassi, 1978). To further research, standardised tests that attempted to measure the trait, or the different aspects, of assertiveness were developed, including both questionnaires and other assessment techniques such as observed role-plays. There are about fifteen of these assessments and Galassi and Galassi (1978) review the majority in their critical analysis of assertion.

Another way of measuring assertiveness has been through behavioural assessment, by observing the subject's behaviour either in a simulated or a natural setting. The most popular technique is role-play, having others rate observable behaviours, such as speech and eye-contact.

In terms of the assessment of assertion to date, efforts to validate assessments to high standards of reliability have so far been limited. In addition, little regard has been taken of the meaning of assertiveness for different areas of the population. It is also apparent from the psychological research literature that more qualitative/clinical descriptive studies are needed.

Assertiveness and related concepts

So far, assertiveness has been described as a set of skills that can be measured, and if lacking can be acquired. However, the role that assertiveness plays in the general psychological well-being and functioning of the whole person is also of significance. Once the skills are acquired, the assertive person can allow the expression of parts of their personality that may previously have been hidden, or at least inhibited. This will have ramifications within the person's whole psychological system and of those around her. For these reasons there are a number of psychological constructs that are necessarily linked with assertion, as demonstrated by the following.

Self-esteem

One frequently cited relationship is that of assertion to self-esteem. Petrie and Rotherham (1982) examined the links between self-esteem, assertiveness, and stress, using self-report measures to assess these three. The findings indicated that self-esteem and assertiveness are significantly and inversely related to stress, with assertiveness contributing to self-esteem, and self-esteem being directly linked to stress. The conclusion was that AT could be used as a means of increasing self-esteem, and so indirectly decreasing stress. Shafer (1988) found similar results when looking at the relationship between equality and inequality, self-esteem, and happiness; it may be presumed that assertiveness may have a fundamental effect on the equality displayed within a relationship.

Anxiety

That stress and anxiety are related to both mental and physical health is clear (Baum and Singer, 1987). From the literature reviewed it is also clear that stress and anxiety are negatively related to assertive behaviour. How AT can be used to reduce stress, and to help with other problems such as depression will be reviewed in a later section.

Anxiety is central to unassertiveness in two different ways. Firstly, it is one reason why a non-assertive response is made in the first place, that is, to escape an anxiety-provoking situation. This type of response, however, does not change anything, and it is likely that the person will repeatedly find themselves in anxiety-provoking situations. Secondly, the long-term effects of behaving in a nonasssertive way have detrimental effects upon self-esteem, and so on, and further increase inhibition and impede self-expression. The culminating effect of this is an increased distance between the ideal self and the real self, leading to increased levels of stress and anxiety. An increase in assertive behaviour may lead to an initial, temporary, context specific heightening of anxiety, but in the long-term the amelioration of situations that provoke anxiety, plus great self-fulfilment in terms of realising one's potential, leads to more positive experiences and less stress and anxiety.

Self-concept

Percell and Berwick (1974) related AT to self-concept and anxiety. Again the findings substantiate the hypothesis that anxiety can be reduced by the use of AT to increase self concept. This study also identified that a strong, significant relationship existed between assertion and anxiety measures for women only, indicating that assertive women are significantly less anxious than unassertive women.

Self-actualisation

Looking back at the early theories of assertion, self-actualisation was frequently seen as a working element within a more complex and sophisticated system, such as Maslow's self-actualisation hierarchy (1970). Crandall *et al.* (1988) demonstrated that AT significantly increased self-actualisation, for at least one year, and the longer-term improvements were only slightly less than the immediate change on completion of the course. Olzak and Goldman (1981) also found a significant relationship between assertiveness and self-actualisation, and go on to comment that, 'The findings of a high positive relationship between self-actualisation (psychological health) and assertiveness is consistent with the theorizing of Maslow (1970) and the recent trend of viewing assertiveness training within a "health" model orientation.'

Self-empowerment

This concept also has its roots in Maslow's hierarchy of needs (1970) and also draws upon other work, such as that of Ellis's 'Rational Emotive Therapy'. In today's society the idea of self-empowerment underpins such developments as consciousness-raising within the women's movement, and self-advocacy within groups of people with disabilities. The theory states that the traditional life-style imposes 'oughts' and 'shoulds' upon the person that conflict or create tension between their inner needs and wishes (Forester, 1977). The idea of the traditional life-style can be linked with the concept of socialisation, by which values and ideals are imposed and imprinted upon the individual through their social experience. Judge (1985), in her description of the self-empowerment theory, indicates the different dimensions involved in the concept such as awareness, purpose, concepts, skills and information; all components vital to most AT packages.

Locus of control

Locus of control deserves particular mention because of its close association with health, health education, and health-care theory, in addition to the abundance of research material upon the topic. Rotter (1966) introduced the concept of locus of control, which developed out of social learning theory. He suggested two polar 'ends' to the concept: 'internals' being those people who have a general expectation that positive and/or negative events are under their control; 'externals', on the other hand, have a general expectation that events are unrelated to their behaviour.

This theory has important implications for both preventive medicine and health education. Whether one accepts responsibility for one's health is partly dependent upon one's views on the determinants of health and illness. Pill and Stott (1985) show some very interesting findings within a sample of working-class mothers on a suburban housing estate:

> We found that at least half the sample held fatalistic views about illness causation, i.e. they subscribed to theories which regarded the causation of illness as external to the individual and hence outside individual control. These women were prepared to accept the concept of blame, the notion that sometimes people may have themselves to blame if they fell ill, under very restricting circumstances involving direct risk taking. The remainder of the sample were prepared to recognise that individual behaviour had some part to play in illness causation and they were more likely to accept that neglect of oneself could reduce the level of resistance to illness.
>
> This broad division in the nature of health beliefs appeared to relate to the amount of formal education the women had received; the greater the amount the nearer the respondents were to official views on effective ways of maintaining health.

Further studies have examined locus of control in relation to specific health behaviours, for example weight loss, smoking, alcohol abuse, and medical compliance, such as in diabetes and hypertension. Judge (1985) provides a review of some of these areas, as well as psychological/ psychiatric issues such as depression and stress. Locus of control seems to have importance in most of these areas in terms of health care, however no generalisations can be made because the influence of locus of control may vary depending on the topic. Nevertheless there remains much interest in locus of control in terms of modifying the way that people think about health and illness, in order to promote change in health behaviour.

Tanck and Robbins (1979) demonstrated that people who are assertive have a more internal view of control than those who are not assertive. In investigating the link between assertiveness, locus of control, and health, Williams and Stout (1985) hypothesised that 'highly assertive individuals would report significantly fewer health problems and significantly greater internal control than would those low in assertiveness' and indeed their findings confirmed this.

Self-efficacy

The concept of self-efficacy is receiving increasing attention as a predictor of health behaviour change and maintenance (Strecher *et al.*, 1986). Bandura (1977) differentiates between locus of control and self-efficacy in that the former is a generalised concept about oneself, and the latter is situation-specific – focused on beliefs about one's abilities to behave in certain ways in specific settings, which would often include interpersonal interactions. People who regard outcomes as personally determined but who lack the requisite skills would experience low self-efficacy, and approach activities with a sense of futility. Rosenstock *et al.*, (1988) argue that self-efficacy should be incorporated into the Health Belief Model (Becker, 1974) as a predictor of health behaviour. Rosenstock *et al.* (1988) point out that, 'The problems involved in modifying life-long habits of eating, drinking, exercising and smoking are obviously far more difficult to surmount than are those for accepting a one-time immunisation or screening test. It requires a good deal of confidence that one can in fact alter such lifestyles . . . thus people must feel competent (self-efficacious) to change.'

As will be demonstrated, AT is effective in increasing self-confidence in particular situations. Anxiety results when people see themselves as ill-equipped to deal with potentially damaging events, and anxiety in turn may influence expectations of efficacy. Since AT is a technique that aims to reduce anxiety levels by improving the skills required to handle such situations, it clearly has enormous potential for enhancing self-efficacy in health behaviours that require effective interpersonal interactions.

In a comprehensive review of studies linking self-efficacy to behaviour in the areas of smoking, weight control, alcohol abuse, exercise and contraception, Strecher *et al.* (1986), found that in all these areas, self-efficacy was a consistent predictor of short- and long-term success. In experimental studies, manipulations of self-efficacy have proven consistently powerful in initiating and maintaining change. The methods used in these studies and in AT both involve the development of an awareness of the behaviour required in specific situations, through techniques such as rehearsal, modelling, anxiety-control techniques, and verbal reinforcement. Successive mastery over tasks requiring specific behaviour helps the person to develop and refine skills.

What is assertiveness training?

> Assertion training is not a standard technique but a loose amalgamation of a variety of techniques. (Galassi and Galassi, 1978)

> Assertion training is a communication skill which teaches individuals to directly and honestly express their feelings, opinions, thoughts and beliefs. (Del Greco, 1980)

Del Greco (1980) differentiates between two key phases in AT. The first involves the promotion of a value system based on the values held collectively by society, such as the right to be treated with respect; the right to express your feelings; the right to ask for what you want; the right to say 'no' without feeling guilty; the right to give and receive compliments; the right not to fulfil another's expectations of you.

The second phase involves learning the behavioural skills that typify assertive behaviour. Del Greco (1986) describes this as direct eye-contact, conversational voice level, direct posture, positive statements, and direct responses to situations.

Most AT is conducted in a group setting over a number of weeks. Common elements include behaviour rehearsal; modelling; coaching; performance feedback, sometimes using tapes; self-evaluation; reinforcement; practice; instruction; discrimination training; cognitive restructuring, etc., as well as discussion (Rathus, 1973).

What are the aims of assertiveness training?

The goals of most training will probably include: reducing anxiety and fear; changing attitudes and beliefs; aiding motivation; building self-esteem and confidence; and learning new skills and behaviours. 'For me, assertiveness training offers hope. Because it is based on self-esteem, it offers a new way of relating to other people. It has grown with me from a set of communication skills to certain beliefs which are very important to me personally' (Dickson, 1988). Dickson indicates that the women who came to her classes came because they wanted to change their lives in some way: 'A few came to the classes with a clearly defined goal, but most . . . were pushed by some dimly-felt awareness that all was not well in their lives. Many felt that they lacked control over their lives. There were a few good days in their lives when they felt confident and secure but mostly they worried . . .' She links these feelings with the benefits of AT by stating that:

'Identifying the circumstances in which you would like to respond differently is an excellent first step towards achieving change in your life.'

In a study to ascertain the current extent and range of assertiveness activities, Whitehead (1990) collected information from a variety of organisations and individuals offering AT, which provides a qualitative overview of current work in this country.

In response to the question regarding the main aims and objectives of the training offered, of 65 replies only eight gave a specific health objective, e.g. reducing stress or anxiety. (The interrelationship between health and many of the other aims mentioned below have already been described). Almost half (31) said the AT they offered was aimed at building women's self-confidence, and 15 referred to enhancing self-esteem specifically or in related terms, such as valuing self, self-respect, etc. Twenty-one referred to promoting awareness of what assertive behaviour is and how it differs from other ways of relating, and to developing these skills. Thirteen included specific reference to personal development in some shape or form; 11 referred to communication skills, and several specifically mentioned improving interpersonal relationships. Nine referred to choice, control, goal-setting or decision-making, and taking personal responsibility for these.

In contrast to these broad goals, more specific behavioural objectives were mentioned less frequently: knowing and asserting your rights featured in only four responses; giving and receiving criticism in five; saying 'no' in eight; and dealing with specific difficult situations in 11. Eight referred to improved confidence in dealing with professionals, using services effectively, and so on. In addition, seven specifically identified the opportunity for support and space in which to discuss all of these things, and several referred to the benefits of the changes in women's lives that result from AT not only for the individual, but also for the wider community.

The aims and objectives of AT are thus no longer limited to a purely behaviourist outcome, within interpersonal interactions, but, in response to women's needs and experiences, are being extended to encompass a far wider approach to a better and healthier way of life. It is thus vitally important to recognise that women are redefining the concept of assertiveness in their own terms, as well as recognising the relevance of AT to their lives, health, and well-being on a wide scale. It is also crucial to understand and remember this when considering the relationship of assertiveness to health, and the benefits of AT as a tool for health educators and promoters in a wide variety of settings. The development of assertive behavioural skills instead of passive, aggressive, or manipulative behaviour, however, remains the central focus of AT.

Is AT effective?

In a critical and wide-ranging review of assertion, Galassi and Galassi (1978) indicated that there was a considerable body of evidence for the effectiveness of AT in behavioural psychology. Since then, as the popularisation of AT has taken it outside the clinical sphere, there have been fewer studies measuring the effectiveness of the broader approaches described earlier. Furthermore the community focus means that AT's virtues are more likely to be extolled in the popular press than in academic journals. Certainly the popularity it has achieved speaks for itself.

In any case evaluation is difficult since AT is not a unique or even well-defined behavioural training process. It is a complex, unsystematic, and unstandardised procedure that uses a variety of techniques (Rich, 1976). Despite this, a number of studies have examined whether AT groups have improved assertiveness skills as well as other psychological attributes such as self-esteem, in comparison to other therapeutic techniques. For example, Lomont *et al.* (1969) compared group AT to group insight-therapies. Using a personality test as an outcome measure they found that at the end of the training there were significant increases in factors related to assertiveness, and a reduction on the scales that related to clinical factors, e.g. anxiety. No such difference was found with the group insight-therapy.

Rathus (1972) compared group AT with discussion groups and a control group. Fifty-seven female students were randomly assigned to the three types of group, which met once a week for seven weeks. Rathus's assertiveness schedule was used as an outcome measure. As a further means of evaluation, videotaped role-plays were used that were then rated by independent raters. The results showed that the difference in gains between the AT and the control subjects was highly significant. AT subjects also reported greater reduction in the fear they experienced during social confrontations than did those in the discussion or control group.

Giesen (1988) examined whether the initial gains made in an AT group were maintained over a period of time. She stresses the importance of finding out if the new behaviour is maintained because it can then be speculated that internal reinforcers have been established in the person that alone are sufficient to reinforce the assertive behaviour, or that the new behaviour has caused changes in the person's environment such that both external and internal reinforcers now encourage assertiveness. A health checklist demonstrated differences approaching significance in health status, with the AT group showing fewer health problems than prior to joining the group, in contrast to the comparison group, which reported more health problems. In addition, the training group women were interviewed after the close of the group:

The women reported positive changes in self-attitudes, self-confidence and ease of expressing themselves, and felt less anxiety or discomfort in social situations or in meeting new people . . .

Positive reactions from others and rewarding situational changes were reported by six women as occurring early in the course, while the remaining five women reported positive reactions occurring later during or after training. (Giesen, 1988)

The positive changes included successful negotiation for more assistance from partners, more free time for independent activities, and better communication with partners, employers, and children. This is a particularly significant study because the women involved were not college students or in contact with the psychiatric service systems, but white, middle-class women who simply wished to improve their assertiveness skills.

Kincaid (1978) followed up a group AT course over a two-year period. The 60 respondents ranged in age from 22–63 years (mean age 31); all were middle-class, and all but three were white. The results showed an enthusiastic response to the course, and increased assertiveness in interpersonal relationships. They also showed that the women felt their work had only just started, and that they needed to develop further before their desired level of assertiveness would be reached. In addition, many requested further training, either generally or focused on specific topics, such as interpersonal and sexual relationships.

An interesting variation to the usual group training or one-to-one approach to AT is self-study (for example, see Lindenfield, 1986). An up-to-date bibliography including a number of such books is incorporated into Whitehead's (1990) report. Surprisingly, the effectiveness of these guides and self-help methods has not been systematically researched, and remains a possibly fruitful area of study.

One study that addresses a similar issue is that of Kann (1987), who demonstrated that a computer-assisted instruction programme used in schools increased assertiveness knowledge and behaviour for both females and males in relation to responsible sexuality. Decision-making knowledge and behaviour, and interpersonal communication knowledge were also found to have increased.

Part Two
Links between assertiveness and health – How AT can promote women's health

This section develops the links between assertiveness and health, focusing on women's health and on the demonstrable benefits of AT on various aspects of women's health. Finally, it looks at issues involving AT for particular population groups.

The effect of socialisation on assertiveness and other aspects of women's health

It is important to address why women in particular consider themselves, and are considered to be, in need of AT.

Holandsworth and Wall (1977) found that on self-report measures of assertion, 'without exception' males reported higher frequencies of assertive behaviour than females. However, there were some interesting differences in the areas where assertiveness was exhibited. For example, men tend to be more assertive in relating to bosses and supervisors, being outspoken when stating opinions, and taking the initiative in social contact with the opposite sex. Women tend to be more assertive in expressing love and affection, compliments, and in expressing anger with parents.

Arguments explaining this gender difference originate from two different directions: firstly, the view that women are socialised into being less assertive than men; and secondly, that women face particular stresses as a consequence of their gender, in addition to the consequences of being generally more passive than men.

There is much support for the contention that women are socialised early and throughout their lives into adopting different social roles to men (Williams, 1987). For example, Kagan and Moss (1962) found that parents and teachers permitted and encouraged aggression in small boys in contrast to dependency and passivity in girls. Hence adult women are consistently characterised as less aggressive, more passive, and more submissive than men (Rosenkrantz *et al.*, 1968; Broverman *et al.*, 1970; Spence *et al.*, 1974). Studies have also shown that women frequently see themselves as less aggressive than men (Buss, 1961; Lowenstein, 1977), and report feeling guilt at behaving aggressively (Sears, 1961). Passivity is also linked to poor self-confidence, lowered self-esteem, fear of success, and impaired personal and professional relationships (Moore, 1979). Wolf and Fodor (1975) summarise the effects of sex-role socialisation as follows:

> . . . for males, socialisation tends to enhance experimental options . . . the male socialisation experience involves learning to be assertive, competitive, independent, aggressive; for females the socialization process tends to reinforce the nurturant, docile, submissive and conservative aspects of the traditionally defined female role and discourages personality qualitites conventually defined as masculine; self-assertiveness, achievement orientation, and independence. It is largely through nurturant, docile programming of the female role that women in particular seem to end up with such severe deficits in assertive behaviour.

It is not hard to see why women frequently adopt a nonassertive role, which, as we have demonstrated, often leads to deleterious psychological consequences. For example, it has been found that women suffer greater depression (Weisman and Klerman, 1978) and other forms of mental illness than do men (Chesler, 1972). Indeed, 36% of women were found to suffer stress very or quite often, compared with 25% of men (BRMB statistics, 1989). Many of these women reported responding to stress by drinking alcohol, smoking, or arguing.

Sex-role socialisation in itself has generalised and far-reaching effects, encompassing other psychological characteristics in addition to assertion, and being found to exert additional stress on women (Moore, 1979). Wark (1980), in her review of the effects of gender-role stereotyping and the effects on women's health notes that, 'The more social emphasis there is on culturally-defined rather than sex-linked behaviours, the more likely it is that stress will be introduced into individuals, male or female, as they will more frequently fail to conform to the cultural expectations of the society.'

Ray and Lovejoy (1984) found that 'femininity' correlated strongly with a lack of assertiveness and a lack of self-esteem. A rigid masculine orientation, however, also went with low self-esteem and low assertiveness. Such rigidity also militates against the possibility of individuals attaining a strongly perceived internal locus of control, being able to take responsibility for their health, restrict choice, and inhibit achievement of self-actualisation. This limitation of personal development is clearly unhealthy: '. . . any form of stereotyping restricts individual freedom and choice and so can be considered to be socially or psychologically unhealthy' (Wark, 1980).

The social and cultural factors which work to maintain traditional sex-role stereotyping include both negative attitudes and structural constraints, and are incorporated in the concept of 'sexism'. It is not hard to imagine the stress resulting for those women who try and break out of the expected passive role, and the additional problems posed for those women who attempt to swim against the powerful social tide. Carlyon (1981) identified this as an issue for health educators when he wrote:

> I was struck by how little attention health education pays to sexism as a health problem. There is no social force more destructive of personal growth and fulfilment than institutionalised prejudice, of which sexism and racism are leading examples. Surely systematic humiliation and degradation deserve as much attention as barriers to achieving health as do poor eating habits and sloth.

AT can plan a key role in enabling women to break out of stifling, inflexible, and passive roles resulting in boundless improvements in health. Lirette (1979) studied the interrelationship between assertiveness, self-actualisation, psychopathology, and sex-role socialisation. Her findings confirmed that higher levels of assertiveness were associated with lower levels of psychopathology. She concluded that, 'The data clearly show that for males being assertive is healthy and integrated into what it means to be male in this culture . . . The finding that assertiveness is positively related to self-actualisation affirms the value of learning assertive behaviour as a means for increasing psychological health.'

Women's health issues

Following the pattern of growth in the United States, and paralleling the growth of women's interest in health, AT as a way of increasing women's confidence has grown in popularity in the last two decades in Britain. While women's concerns with, and involvement in, health are long-standing, in recent years the focus has been concerned with increasing choice and facilitating access to those options:

> Health in its broadest meaning was central to many of the questions raised, linked as it was to a woman's sense of herself and her right to make choices, in terms of both personal relationships and public life. Women and health groups were concerned to redefine women as 'healthy', to demystify medical knowledge and to make it more widely available. (WEA, 1988)

The right to choice and control – in sexuality, birth control, fertility, childbirth, and medical treatment – and a desire to alter imbalances in power relationships between women and men, women and the medical profession, and between health workers, were central themes. The contribution AT can make to achieving these aims is obvious.

Reagan, writing in 1981, made the parallels between the women's health movement and health education explicit:

> When one reads of preventive health concepts, self-awareness or personal control, the likelihood is that one would think these to be definitions of health education. Interestingly these terms also describe the rebirth of another important program, the women's health movement. The rejuvenation of the women's health movement and the growing credibility of the self-care movement deserve to be viewed for what they are – important, although neglected, parts of health education . . . above all, health education can do for women what it does best for all. It can help people feel good about their ability to be themselves, to feel normal and distinctive, to have

a sense of self that allows for positive decision-making and self-actualised behaviour.

There are several important messages here for health educators. Women's experience of health and well-being is often less related to those aspects commonly used as measures of health by people who are planning services, whether preventive, educational, or curative. Women are redefining their experience of health, and equating their health with the control they have over their lives and choices about health care, and equally, health behaviours.

Choi (1985) argues for a new paradigm for women's health care: 'Overall goals would include the development or enhancement of a sense of dignity and responsibility within the individual – assisting women to become knowledgeable about the processes and events that affect their health and nurturing confidence in their ability to make changes that will improve their health.'

Thus to promote women's health is to facilitate choice, which can be viewed on a number of levels: first, at an informational level, to be aware of choice and information about options available; second, to have the decision-making skills required to set goals and ascertain appropriate courses of action to achieve them; third, to have the self-confidence and self-esteem to believe one has the right to make such choices; fourth, the ability to carry out these choices, which usually involves making them known to, understood and respected by and adhered to by others. All of these stages are involved in social and life-skills training, and specifically in AT. All these stages require assertive behaviour, self-respect, self-esteem, and self-confidence, therefore it is clear that AT offers a positive approach to better health for women.

How does increasing assertion skills affect health?

There now follow some examples from the literature that demonstrate the relationship between AT and specific health concerns. The sparsity of evaluation of AT with 'well' adults in community settings in relation to health issues is particularly obvious at this point, and so the evidence in this section rests largely on patient- and schools-based studies.

Smoking

AT has been shown to be useful in the area of addictive behaviour. Del Greco (1980) designed an AT programme aimed at preventing smoking by adolescents, on the basis of the considerable evidence that adolescents who smoke are more vulnerable to peer pressure and have a higher level of conformity than nonsmokers (Price, 1973; Zagona *et al.*, 1965; Schnieder, 1974; Lanesee, 1972; Roberts *et al.*, 1970; and Salber, 1963, 1971). She argued that since the peer group is essential to the adolescent life-style, it is imperative that adolescents learn how to express themselves and follow their own convictions – in this case to remain a nonsmoker – and yet not alienate themselves from their peer group. Since assertive behaviour is a communication skill based upon the expression of thoughts and feelings, enabling the person to stand up for their rights without violating the rights of others or without leading to alienation, Del Greco believed that AT would achieve this aim.

She designed a course in which situations related to cigarette smoking would be introduced, role-played, and discussed, such as refusing a cigarette from a friend, refusing to pool money to buy cigarettes, or asking someone not to smoke near you. In evaluating this work after a four-year period, Del Greco (1986) found that while assertion did not predict smoking behaviour at the pre-test, there was a gradation in smoking at the post-test. The lowest levels of smoking were in the group receiving AT alongside an innovative smoking education programme; higher in the smoking programme only; and highest in the control group, although differences were not statistically significant.

Recent work by Hynes (1989) developed this theme by including the teaching of social skills and behaviours which could help young people to resist initiating smoking, by such activities as AT through role-play. Botvin (1989) identified a low level of assertiveness as one of a constellation of personality variables, including heavier alcohol usage, which was a predictor of adolescents using 'smokeless tobacco'.

Botvin's earlier work (1980) showed that a life-skills approach to the prevention of cigarette smoking in young people, including work on self-image, coping with anxiety, communication and social skills, and AT, led to significant differences in the proportion of 'new' experimental smokers between the experimental and control groups.

Alcohol

Similar work by Botvin (1984) around alcohol education demonstrated that personal and social-skills training, including decision-making, coping with anxiety, general social skills and assertiveness (including techniques for resisting peer pressure to drink), led to a significantly greater proportion of the students in the experimental group drinking less frequently, drinking less per occasion, and less frequent episodes of drunkenness compared with a control group.

Rohrbach *et al.* (1987) used resistance-skills training – a specific aspect of assertiveness – in a schools-based alcohol-use prevention programme. Responses were rated on levels of confidence, assertiveness, and nonverbal responses. Students in the test-group performed better on alcohol refusal skills, and showed greater refusal self-efficacy than did students receiving other preventive curricula.

Hirsche *et al.* (1978) set up a controlled study of two experimental groups of alcohol abusers, one receiving 'regular' therapy and the other receiving 10 hours of AT. Their findings supported their hypothesis that group-AT was an effective therapeutic technique for people with serious alcohol problems.

Botvin's pioneering work in the United States in smoking and alcohol education, and Hopson's and Scally's (1979, 1981) equivalent work in this country in developing the comprehensive life-skills teaching programme, has since formed the basis for much current health education work in schools, as referred to in the introduction.

Eating

Several studies support the contention that AT can be valuable in achieving weight loss. McMillan (1975) concluded from an experimental comparison study that a combination of behavioural procedures – including AT, thought-stopping, covert assertion, contingency management, and self-monitoring – can be successful in producing weight loss. Conoley's (1976) study of 20 unassertive overweight women indicated that AT increased assertive behaviour, altered food intake patterns, and lowered anxiety.

Sexual health

Kann (1987) identifies assertiveness, decision-making, and interpersonal communication as basic interaction skills underlying responsible sexual behaviour. Yet a survey (Holland, 1990) of the first sexual experiences of 150 women aged between 16 and 21 showed that many teenage girls having sex for the first time do so reluctantly because they do not have the power to resist. Because the girls lack the power to control these encounters, they also lack control over protection, and are exposed to the risk of AIDS, other infections, and pregnancy. The authors conclude: 'We must try and empower women with information about relationships, emotions and feelings. Health education policy will be ineffective if the imbalance of power is not understood and acted upon.'

Working with adolescents, Gilchrist and Schinke (1983) combined factual information with skills training and practice, including the initiation of discussion of birth control, the acquisition of contraception, and the refusal of unacceptable demands. Subsequently students showed marked improvements in efficacy ratings of their own abilities to use birth control, exhibited more effective contraception-solving abilities, and had greater intentions of using contraception at next intercourse than did a group of students not receiving the intervention.

Menopause

Bart and Perlmutter (1981) cite cross-cultural research that suggests that depression during menopause is not so much related to physiological changes as to social and cultural factors, and that lack of self-esteem seems to account for the incidence of menopausal depression. The transition to the nonreproductive years is harder for women giving up the highly valued role of mothering. Women who are low in self-esteem and life satisfaction may be most likely to have a difficult menopause. It is not surprising that AT is increasingly recommended as an important part of a self-help strategy for menopausal women (Rakusen, 1989; Lindeman, 1984) or incorporated as a key element in a comprehensive course for such women, for example The City and Hackney Well-Women Centre ran four successful menopause support-groups with a key assertiveness element, alongside work on validation of self and self-image (Cosgrove, 1989).

Pelvic pain

AT was part of a package which was used to assist women who were suffering undiagnosed, chronic, pelvic pain (Petrucco and Harris, 1982). Using relaxation and counselling aimed at increasing the women's assertiveness, 11 of the 16 women not having a hysterectomy were found either to have improved or to have been pain-free after a six-month follow-up.

Duodenal ulcer

Stress and anxiety are clearly indicated in ulcer etiology and exacerbation (Minski and Desai, 1955). Gildea (1949) suggested that ulcer patients also exhibit tendencies to inhibit repression of negative emotions, to over-conform, and to be nonassertive. Consequently, Brooks (1980) used emotional-skills training with a group of patients who had X-ray confirmation of uncomplicated duodenal ulcer. AT, together with anxiety management, led to significant decreases in symptomatology for all patients, with less pain and more rapid healing. Furthermore, it significantly reduced the recurrence rate of duodenal ulcer three-and-a-half years after the intervention, compared with an attention placebo treatment group. This study illustrates in a measurable way the effectiveness of AT in reducing stress, and hence one of its possible physiological consequences.

Mental health

As already demonstrated, assertiveness, or lack of it, is closely related to attributes such as self-esteem, self-confidence, and self-actualisation, which in turn are all important components of mental health. Furthermore, there is a close relationship between lack of assertiveness and specific mental health problems as illustrated below.

Anxiety and stress

That anxiety and general mental stress are extremely deleterious to both physical and psychological health is now
well accepted (Baum and Singer, 1987). It follows that
increasing assertiveness skills will reduce stress and
anxiety, so ultimately helping to maintain good health.
Percell and Berwick (1974) studied the effects of AT on
both anxiety and self-concept. The study found a strong
relationship between anxiety and assertion: the less
assertive the person, the more anxious they are likely to
be. This relationship was found to exist only for women.
After eight group sessions, the participants who increased in assertiveness also became more self-accepting
and less anxious.

Sedgewick *et al.* (1989) carried out a much larger study
involving 595 men and women over a one-to-seven-year
period, looking at the effects of a stress-management
course that had an AT component. Although confounded
with the other components of the stress inoculation
course (rational thinking, priority-setting, relaxation training), the results indicated a substantial reduction in
perceived stress, even after follow-up. These and other
studies clearly verify the link between AT and the reduction of stress.

Anger

Other aspects of psychological health have been examined
in relation to assertion skills that have a bearing on physical
health, for example anger control, which is directly
linked to physical conditions such as heart disease. It has
been found that individuals who tend to suppress hostile
emotions rather than express them in an appropriate
way have altered blood pressure levels, which in the long
term were found to be deleterious to their health
(Gambarro and Rabin, 1969). It also has been found that
sex-role socialisation is a potent determinant in the

expression of anger (Broverman and Broverman, 1968). In a study examining sex-role stereotypy, anger expression, and psychosomatic symptoms, Heiser and Gannon (1984) found that people who were both unassertive and repressed their anger reported more health problems.

Depression

Depression is also related to assertiveness. Sanchez and Lewinsohn, working in the United States, have looked specifically at this area with some interesting findings (Sanchez and Lewinsohn, 1979; Sanchez, Lewinsohn and Larson, 1980). Earlier work (Lazarus, 1972) had suggested there was a negative correlational link between assertion and depression. However, it was unclear whether less assertive individuals were more susceptible to depression, or whether depression made individuals less assertive. Sanchez *et al.*'s (1979, 1980) work attempted to examine this question. Their 1979 study used a five-week AT course and measured through daily self-report measures both the level of depression and the rate of assertive behaviours. They found that low levels of assertive behaviour were a better predictor of subsequent levels of depression than depression was a predictor of unassertive behaviour. They went on to conclude that therapeutic interventions that increase levels of assertive behaviour may prove useful in the treatment of depression.

In a later study, Sanchez *et al.* (1980) compared AT with traditional group psychotherapy as a treatment for depression. Thirty-two women were randomly assigned to one of four groups, two AT groups and two psycho-therapy groups. Each group met for 1½ hours, twice weekly, over a five-week period. Interestingly, medication was available as an adjunctive treatment for all patients: the therapists in the AT group voiced opinions against the use of such drugs, the other therapists did not. Ten of the 16 in the psychotherapy groups used drugs ranging from the minor tranquillizers and hypnotics to anti-depressants; none of the participants in the assertion groups used drugs. Assessments of assertion and depression were made using self-report measures, pre-treatment, post-treatment, and at one-month follow-up. At post-treatment the assertion group had made greater improvements on all measures than the psychotherapy group, but this difference was not statistically significant until follow-up. At follow-up the assertion group had continued making progress over the 30-day period, and the differences between treatments were found to be significant for all of the measures used.

Although Sanchez and Lewinsohn express some caution over these results because four therapists were used, undoubtedly introducing variance into the groups, they also make the point that antidepressant medication reduces depressive symptomatology, and since most of those in the psychotherapy group used such drugs, it makes the results of the study even more impressive.

Suicidal behaviour

Studies have shown that firstly, a lack of assertiveness was linked with severe depression and consequent suicidal behaviour, and, secondly, AT was successful in reducing suicidal behaviour.

Sifneos (1970) found that 66% of suicide-attempters were trying to manipulate or control another person, usually their partner, and Fawcett (1966) noted that the majority of his suicidal clients seemed totally unable to communicate to significant individuals exactly what they wanted; they also appeared unable to bargain effectively with their partners. Hattem (1964) found that several of his clients attributed their suicidal feelings to their partner's rejection. In all these cases, increased assertiveness might have facilitated better communication with partners, and hence lessen the cause of the depressive feelings that led to suicide attempts.

Bartman (1976), compared a 12-session AT programme with open discussion groups used as therapy for people admitted to a psychiatric ward for suicide attempts (excluding psychotics and drug and alcohol abusers). The results indicated that AT led to significantly greater changes in assertive behaviour, and also led to a significantly greater reduction in suicidal behaviour than did the discussion groups.

Whereas such application is clearly 'secondary prevention', how much more valuable it would be to make AT widely available, and thus minimise the interpersonal problems that can lead to deep depression and suicidal behaviour.

Other aspects of health

That an increase in a woman's assertiveness skills is beneficial in a holistic way can also be argued on the basis of research findings, e.g. linking employment and health. An increasing number of mothers have been returning to work after the birth of their children and women generally are once again striving to compete with men within the employment market. It is easy to see that for these women to compete successfully they must acquire the assertiveness skills that men have been shown to have (Holandsworth and Wall, 1977); women who are assertive are also more likely to gain employment.

That employment is beneficial to physical health has been demonstrated by Verbrugge (1983), who examined the influence of multiple roles upon the physical health of men and women. Her findings showed that, concerning the three adult roles of employment, marriage and parenthood the men and women who had the best health were those having all three roles; this is also the case for employed, nonmarried mothers. Thus, if assertiveness is going to help women into employment – and it seems sensible that considerable assertiveness skills will be necessary to maintain multiple social roles –

then AT can have directly beneficial effects on women's physical health.

Compliance

While certain forms of behavioural training with patients may be viewed as one form of health education, equally, where adherence to such treatment is necessary to prevent further damage due to the disease, this may be viewed as secondary prevention. For example, the training offered to diabetics in controlling their condition in terms of insulin use, blood testing and dietary control; failure to comply with medical advice may have serious results and may lead to deterioration in their health. In fact, approximately one-half of all patients with chronic disease fail to follow the directives of medical staff (Haynes *et al.*, 1979).

There is already considerable literature on compliance (for a review see Stuart, 1982). Education alone has not been shown to be effective in increasing compliance, and behavioural training, such as self-control skills, has shown more promising results (Bonar, 1977; Rainwater, 1982). Rabin and Amir (1984) found that in diabetics, compliance with treatment and control of their condition could be predicted by their level of assertiveness skills. This was particularly the case in their ability to handle criticism and initiate interactions, including cognitive coping skills such as their ability to view criticism as constructive, and not to lose self-esteem when criticised.

Rabin and colleagues (1986) subsequently devised and tested a programme which aimed to improve overall cognitive and assertiveness skills in general life; application of these skills to the staff–patient interaction; reduction of anxiety through the use of these skills; and eventual compliance to health-care team directives.

The test group consisted of nine women with juvenile diabetes, all with a long history of noncompliance. A range of issues emerged during the group's work, including the negative effects of staff and the women's families' attitudes towards them, and fear of revealing their condition to others.

The group was successful in achieving its objectives – all members reported using the skills in their daily lives and in interaction with staff. Compliance was increased in two ways, firstly, six members dieted and achieved weight loss, and secondly, they also achieved better blood sugar tests. It was emphasised that the mutual support given by group members was crucial in motivational terms.

The study confirms that behavioural and cognitive skills are preventive tools that can be used in a wide variety of stressful situations, and can give a sense of competence to demoralised patients. The authors recommend that by focusing on the links between assertiveness, coping skills, and compliant behaviour, workers can establish group programmes that increase both compliance and confidence (Rabin *et al.*, 1986).

Patient participation

AT can also be used to provide the skills for meaningful and equal communication with the health-care staff, in which the patient is able to express their needs, feelings, and desired outcomes. For example Rogers (1979) demonstrated that, '. . . a good childbirth experience appears to be more related to how fully a woman participates in the experience and to how women make their own decisions, than how easy the birth is, how long or short the labour is, or even where the birth takes place.'

Morford (1984), suggested that unnecessary Caesarean births could be forestalled by changes in the knowledge and behaviours of parturient women. Survey data indicated that:

The best predictor of vaginal birth seemed to be high desire to learn self-assertion, high knowledge of informed consent, low trust and non-compliant behaviour. Conversely, women who reported low desire to assert themselves, high trust in the health care professional, low knowledge of informed consent and compliant behaviour reported significantly higher incidence of Caesarian births.

While these findings must be viewed in the context of the different system of health care in the United States and the high incidence of Caesarean births there, Britain has one of the highest levels of technological intervention in childbirth in Western Europe, as well as the highest rate of stillbirths and deaths of babies in the first week of life (Wesson, 1988). It may therefore be appropriate to incorporate AT into antenatal education in order to facilitate a more active role by women in the birth process. Indeed, Wesson's book (1988) encourages women to make assertive choices in pregnancy and birth so they can retain control over what happens to themselves, which is so vital to their self-esteem as mothers.

Another example is that of the addiction to medically prescribed drugs, which is a major health problem among women (Halas, 1979; Damman and Soler, 1979). Lindemann (1984) argues that the widespread prescription of drugs to women is the outcome of a health-care model that does not recognise or systematically cultivate self-determination as an essential component of health (she defines self-determination as the ability to make decisions and participate in the helping process). She argues for a change from derogatory attitudes and treatment that may be harmful to women, to positive attitudes and treatments in which women are part of the decision-making process about their lives and health.

Many women choose AT as a means of improving their communication with a range of service providers. Often with the specific aim of increasing control over their own health care by improving communication and establishing a more equal partnership with health-care professionals.

It is clear that increasing assertiveness can improve women's health in a vast number of ways, both in relation to increased choice and control in terms of specific behaviours (such as use of contraception, avoiding alcohol, or participation in health care), and also in general terms (such as reduction of anxiety, increase in self-esteem and self-confidence).

Links between assertiveness and health in particular population groups

As AT research that has not been based on the psychiatrically ill population has tended to have been done on college students, a considerable amount of data has been collected about predominantly white, young, middle-class people; there is thus a shortage of data on other sections of the community. However, where there is a commitment by health educators to work with those groups that are most disadvantaged, most at risk, and with the least previous access to health education, resources, or support, particular attention should be paid to the need to focus on certain groups, for example minority ethnic groups. The following section identifies for consideration some relevant areas in relation to assertiveness and the potential for training.

Race and culture

While the use of cultural and racial variables in the assessment of assertion and AT has not received much attention (Caldwell-Colbert, 1982), we may assume that the race and culture of the receiver and deliverer of an assertive message may affect the nature of an assertive response (Garrison, 1986). Lineberger's (1983) work indicated that both black and white people have a tendency to modify their responses in an interracial situation–both in a negative direction. She also found that black people had more difficulty making positive assertive statements, for example, praise and appreciation, and making requests in both intra- and interracial situations than did white people.

There has been speculation that an assertive response by a black person that might be viewed as appropriate by blacks, might be seen as aggressive by whites (Cheek, 1977). A study by Garrison (1986) indicated that black and white people tend to view certain aspects of black assertive responses differently. In fact, black raters found black assertive responses more aggressive than did white raters, particularly among women. Garrison (1986) suggests that because issues relating to black-versus-white assertiveness are generally not taken into account, AT may fail for some black people where it could have succeeded. It is clear that black AT programmes must have a different focus than traditional AT programmes, and must reflect cultural differences, acknowledge the impact of racism, and place the training within the social and cultural context of black people's lives.

Furnham (1979) found a significant difference in levels of assertiveness between three groups of South African nurses – African, Indian, and European (whites) – who were matched in terms of age, sex, education, occupation, and language competence. The Europeans were the most assertive and the Indians the least. Furnham explains the findings in the context of the positions of the three groups within the socio-political structure of the country, together with the effects of the three individual cultures.

A similar interrelationship is suggested by Loo's (1982) study of 100 Chinese-American women, who generally exhibited low self-esteem and assertiveness, and who were frequently dissatisfied with their traditional role in marriage and with the quality of their lives. There was a high prevalence of mental health problems, particularly depression, anxiety, and psychosomatic disorders, but service utilisation was low. This suggests that services may not be perceived as appropriate to their cultural needs, or that culturally there is a taboo on seeking such services. Preventive work should be a high priority with such a group.

A similar review of 278 Puerto Rican women found a causal model relating acculturation, sex-role traditionalism, assertiveness, and symptoms of mental and physical illness. Correlations showed that second-generation Puerto Rican women, when compared with the first generation, were better educated and less sex-role traditional. As hypothesised, sex-role traditionalism correlated negatively with assertiveness, and assertiveness in turn correlated negatively with symptoms (Soto, 1982). The links between sex-role traditionalism, low self-esteem, low assertiveness and ill-health have already been described.

In terms of flexibility of women's roles, it is possible that the interrelationships illustrated by the American studies also exist among groups of minority ethnic women living in this country, particularly among those from the most restrictive cultures. The particular perspective and needs of women from different racial and cultural backgrounds in relation to assertiveness, health, and other factors including racism, clearly require further attention.

Age

Several pieces of research (Del Greco, 1986; Kann, 1987) that measured levels of assertiveness in young people indicate, firstly, that at age 12 males are more assertive than girls, and, secondly, although there is a 'natural' increase in assertiveness over the next four to five years in both sexes, males retain significantly higher scores. Del Greco (1986) points out therefore that at age 16 – a time of sexual initiations – boys are more able to assert themselves than girls, with obvious consequences. Since girls do not 'catch up' in assertiveness through natural development, it is important not only to offer AT to all young women while they are still at school, but also to older women in the community who did not have the benefit of such techniques during their education.

Social class

The close relationship between assertion and self-esteem has already been identified. Kaplan (1973) predicted that self-esteem would be influenced by interactions between age, sex, and social class. Five hundred people completed a measure of 'self-derogation', the tendency to hold oneself in low self-esteem. While overall there were no sex differences, there were sex differences in certain sub-groups within the sample. Among noncollege grad-uates, 64% of the white women held a poor view of themselves compared with 46% of the men. Among the college edu-cated, only 33% of women had high self-derogation scores, while the figure of 46% for the men remained con-stant between the two groups. The better-educated women had better views of themselves; this finding remained true for black women also. Unfortunately, like the assertiveness research, most work on self-esteem in adults has been done with college students, who are less likely to show sex differences (Fransella, 1977).

This is not to suggest that all working-class women think badly of themselves (Fransella, 1977). Even among women living on welfare, there were sharply contrasting attitudes to the role of women and to their own capabilities (Feldeman, 1973; Bendo, 1973). Nonetheless, there is considerable scope for AT to be developed to meet the particular needs of working-class women, and it should be a priority to promote the widest access poss-ible to AT.

Sexual preference

No research was found specifically comparing levels of assertiveness with sexual preference. However, an abundance of research exists that considers closely linked personality traits and behaviours.

Hopkins's (1969) comparison of a matched group of lesbians and heterosexual women indicated that in general the lesbians were more independent, more resilient, more dominant, more self-sufficient, and more composed than the heterosexual women, attributes that are implicitly linked to a high level of assertiveness. Thompson (1971) found that lesbians rated higher on self-confidence, and Siegelman (1972) confirmed that 'the lesbians are better adjusted in some respects than the heterosexuals.' This view was reaffirmed by a number of other comparison studies (Saghir, 1971; Loney, 1972; Armon, 1960; Freedman, 1968), which are reviewed by Rosen (1974).

Similarly, Freedman (1971) and Weinberg (1974) found that psychological testing could not differentiate homosexual males from heterosexuals, and that the psychological adjustment of those who have accepted their sexual orientation was superior in many cases to most heterosexual males in terms of openness and self-disclosure, self-actualisation, and lack of neurotic tendencies (Lehne, 1974).

The evidence that lesbians and homosexual men score higher on personality traits such as self-confidence than do heterosexuals, may have given the impression that they are so happy, healthy, self-confident and self-empowered that they are all well equipped to deal with societal pressures, and that there is no issue to be talked about in relation to health education. This is not the case however because to achieve this state, a number of phases have to be passed through during which self-identi-

fication and self-acceptance takes place, first inter-
nally, and only later, to a greater or lesser extent,
publically. This process takes time, and it is at this
stage of transition that individuals may be most at
risk of suffering ill-health . . . usually through mental
strain arising from difficulties in accepting an identity which is not valued by society, and fear of rejection by family, friends and colleagues. While leading
to mental breakdown in only the minority of cases,
[Schofield, 1965] these pressures still cause reactions
ranging from irritation and inconvenience to severe
and constant stress arising from feelings of guilt,
fear and frustration – obviously not conducive to
mental or physical health. (Pattenson, 1981)

Increasingly lesbians and homosexual men are replacing
negative self-images with self-acceptance and self-esteem.
Appropriate health education could further assist the
process by facilitating access to reliable information and
help, challenging myths and misconceptions, and provid-
ing assertiveness-based training that focuses on the particular needs of these groups, developing skills in dealing
with conflict or criticism, etc., and in developing confidence and self-esteem.

Disability

Assertiveness, along with self-assurance and self-suffi-
ciency, was one of several key personality factors measured in a study of 61 people with severe musculoskeletal
impairments, which considered the relationship of three
major dimensions of independence – psychological,
social, and functional. It was found that functional
abilities were not signifantly related to levels of psychological and social independence. Those with high social/
psychological independence tended to have more assertive, self-assured, and self-sufficient personalities. They

also tended to have fewer emergency medical needs, were in good health generally, were less likely to smoke, and had had fewer months of formal rehabilitation. They were outgoing, predominantly female, and tended to perceive themselves as independent (Nosek *et al.*, 1987).

Keith (1984) defines the purpose of rehabilitation as facilitating independence, while Troutt (1980) defines independence as 'the ability to assume responsibility for decisions without supervision, while making appropriate use of assistance when it is required.'

The links between assertiveness and decision-making have already been identified. Nosek identifies the implications for those involved in the education, rehabilitation, and care of people with severe disabilities. She argues for an operational definition of independence to be accepted that includes psychological, behavioural, and social dimensions, and for rehabilitation programmes to be assessed on each individual's needs and redesigned accordingly. In view of the key role of assertiveness to psychological and social independence that was demonstrated, AT for people with disabilities offers a huge potential in terms of enhancing their independence, whether their disability is congenital or acquired during childhood or adulthood. Whitehead (1990) found that the potential of AT for women with disabilities was largely untapped.

Conclusions

This paper has identified and discussed the multi-dimensional links and relationships between assertiveness and health in order to validate our belief that AT is relevant and important to all those involved in health education policy and practice, regardless of their approach or philosophy. There are many parallels with life-skills training used extensively in schools, but less evidence that health educators have used the techniques as widely with adult women.

Many examples have been given that link assertiveness, or lack of it, implicitly and explicitly with health, and specifically with women's health. There is also plenty of evidence to indicate that AT is an effective, legitimate, and valid technique that can be used to promote health in a general sense and in relation to specific health behaviours or conditions.

AT is a flexible approach that can be tailored to concentrate on behaviour in a specific context, or broadened to address wider issues in women's lives. AT will enable them to relate and communicate effectively in a range of health-related situations, as well as generally improving their overall mental health, as indicated by reductions in anxiety, anger, and depression, and an increase in self-esteem, self-confidence and aggression, etc. It will also aid general communication, and hence potentially enhance all relationships with partners, family, friends, colleagues, professionals, and all those with whom they come in contact.

There is particular potential for the use of AT with

groups of women who have had limited access to AT, including older women, young women, lesbians, women with disabilities, and black and minority ethnic women. There is also a need for further information about the specific needs and experiences of these groups in relation to assertiveness and health.

The majority of resources available for AT fail to make the links with health, or to use health-related examples. The development of such resources would enable the techniques to be more widely available, for use by a variety of people involved in women's health education. A current HEA project is developing such materials, as described in Appendix A.

Appendix A
The HEA assertiveness and women's health education project

This project began with the appointment of the coordinator in January 1990, and should continue until April 1992 when it is intended to publish and disseminate a resource pack on assertiveness and women's health. The project is funded and managed jointly by the Field Development Division (Women's Health Education) and the AIDS and Sexual Health Programme of the HEA. Day to day management and supervision of the coordinator is provided by the Director of Health Promotion, Sheffield Health Authority.

The purpose of the project is to develop methods of working which specifically link assertiveness to women's health, and from this work to produce resource materials for assertiveness and women's health education. The resources would be suitable in a range of contexts for use by women with experience of AT, who are working with groups of women to promote their health and confidence.

The material will have a particular focus on work with young women, older women, women with disabilities, and black and minority ethnic women, and will incorporate a strong element of sexual health into the overall work. That is, a large component of the work will be enhancing women's skills to enable them to make healthy sexual choices.

A further objective of the project is to monitor and evaluate the effects AT can have on women's health.

Since taking up the post in January 1990, the coordinator

has established a group of 26 women (the facilitators) based in 19 different locations around the country. They include: health workers with both statutory and voluntary agencies, community and youth workers, WEA and further education tutors, a GP and a psychotherapist. The work they are doing for this project forms part of the work which their own organisations fund them to do. Whether the focus of their work was women's health education or AT or both, they all wished to develop the links between the two, and thus contribute to the process of making AT a recognised and valid form of preventative health care.

The group is currently in the process of developing work on confidence, assertiveness, sexual health and women's health generally for the groups with which they work. The facilitators' experience of working with these groups, and the materials that they produce will be collated, coordinated and written up into a draft resource package during the summer of 1991. This will be piloted with further groups of women. modified as necessary, and produced as a resource pack in April 1992.

A report on the development and process of the whole project will also be written, and should be made available by the HEA to stimulate the development of similar projects in the future.

For further information about the HEA Assertiveness and Women's Health Education project please contact the coordinator – Chrissie Whitehead, Burwell House, North Street, Burwell, Cambridge CB5 OBA. Tel: 0638 741256; or Lesley Pattenson, HEA, Hamilton House, Mabledon Place, London WC1H 9TX. Tel: 071 383 3833.

References

Alberti, R. and Emmons, M. (1974) *Your perfect right: a guide to assertive behaviour*, (1st edn). San Luis Obispo, CA: Impact.

Alberti, R. and Emmons, M. (1987) *Your perfect right: a guide to assertive behaviour*, (5th edn). San Luis Obispo, CA: Impact.

Anderson, J. (1986) Health skills: the power to choose. *Health education J.* **45** (1): 19-24.

Anon. (1990) *Health education in schools – a survey of head teachers and health coordinators*. Health Education Authority.

Armon, V. (1960) Some personality variables in overt female homosexuality. *J. of professional and technical personality assessment* **24**: 292-309. (In Rosen, 1974, *op. cit.*)

Bakker, C. and Bakker-Rabdau, M. (1973) *No trespassing: explorations in human territoriality*. San Francisco, CA: Chandler and Sharp.

Bandura, A. (1977) Self-efficacy: towards a unifying theory of behavioural change. *Psychological review* **84**: 191-215.

Barnes, F. (ed.) (1987) *Ambulatory maternal health care and family planning services*. American Public Health Association. (In Choi, 1985, *op. cit.*)

Bart, P. and Perlmutter, E. (1981) *The menopause in changing times*. In Justice, B. and Pore, R. (eds), *The second decade: the impact of the women's movement on American institutions*. Westport, CT: Greenwood Press. (In Lindemann, 1984 *op. cit.*)

Bartman, E.R. (1976) Assertive training with hospitalised suicide attempters. *Dissertation abstracts international* **37** (3): 1425-B.

Baum, A. and Singer, J. (1987) *Handbook of psychology and health*. New York: Laurence Erlbaum.

Becker, M.H. (ed.) (1974) The health belief model and personal health behaviour. *Health education monographs* **2**: 324–473.

Bendo, A. and Feldman, H. (1973) A comparison of the self concept of low-income women with and without husbands present. *Cornell J. of social relations* **9**: 53–85. (In Fransella, 1977, *op. cit.*)

Bonar, J. (1977) *Diabetes: a clinical guide*. New York: Medical Examination Pub. Co. (In Rabin *et al.*, 1986, *op. cit.*)

Botvin, G.J., Eng, A. and Williams, C.L. (1980) Preventing the onset of cigarette smoking through life-skills training. *Preventive medicine* **9**: 135–143.

Botvin, G.J., Baker, E., Botvin, E.M., Filazzola, A.D. and Millman, R.B. (1984) Prevention of alcohol misuse through the development of personal and social competence: a pilot study. *J. of studies in alcohol* **45** (6): 550–552.

Botvin, G.J., Baker, E., Tortu, S., Dusenbury, L. and Gessula, J. (1989) Smokeless tobacco use among adolescents: correlates and concurrent predictors. *J. of developmental and behavioural pediatrics* **10** (4): 181–186.

Brookes, G. and Richardson, F. (1980) Emotional skills training: a treatment programme for duodenal ulcer. *Behaviour therapy* **11**: 198–207.

Broverman, I., Broverman, D., Clarkson, D., Rosenkrantz, P. and Vogel, S. (1970) Sex-role stereotypes and clinical judgements of mental health. *J. of consulting and clinical psychology* **3** (1): 1–7.

Buss, A. (1961) *The psychology of aggression*. New York: John Wiley & Sons.

Caldwell-Colbert, A.T. and Jenkins, J.O. (1982) Modification of interpersonal behaviour. In Turner, S. and Jones, R. (eds), *Behaviour modification in the black populations*, pp. 171–207. New York: Plenum Press. (In Garrison, 1986, *op. cit.*)

Carlyon, W.H. (1981) Letter to the editor. *Health education* **May/June 1981**.

Cheek, D.K. (1976) *Assertive black . . . puzzled white*. San Luis Obispo, CA: Impact.

Chesler, P. (1972) *Women and madness*. New York: Doubleday.

Choi, M.W. (1985) Preamble to a new paradigm for women's health care. *Image: the j. of nursing scholarship* **17**: (1) 14–16.

Conoley, C.W. (1976) The effects of vicarious reinforcement in assertive training on assertive behaviour, anxiety and food intake of underassertive obese females. *Dissertation abstracts international 2497-B*.

Cosgrove, T. (1989) *Menopause groups – the development of a service*. The City and Hackney Health Authority publication.

Crandall, R., McCown, D. and Robbs, Z. (1988) The effects of assertion training on self-actualisation. *Small group behaviour* **19** (1): 134–145.

Dammam, G. and Soler, E. (1979) Prescription drug abuse: a San Francisco study. *Frontiers* **4**: 5–10. (In Lindemann, 1984, *op. cit.*)

Del Greco, L. (1980) Assertiveness training for adolescents: a potentially useful tool in the prevention of cigarette smoking. *Health education J.* **39** (3): 80–82.

Del Greco, L., Breitbach, L., Rumer, S., McCarthy, R.H. and Suissa, S. (1986) Four-year results of a youth smoking prevention program using assertiveness training. *Adolescence* **21** (83): 631–640.

Dickson, A. (1982, 1988 edns) *A woman in your own right – assertiveness and you*. London: Quartet Books. (Revd edn 1988.)

Dollard, J. and Miller, N.E. (1950) *Personality and psychotherapy*. New York: McGraw-Hill. (In Rathus, 1975, *op. cit.*)

Dua, J. and McNall, H. (1987) Assertiveness in men and women seeking counselling and not seeking counselling. *Behaviour change* **4** (1): 14–19.

Fawcett, J.A. (1966) Newer developments in psycho-pharmacology and therapy in depression. In *Depression and suicide*, Vermont Department of Mental Health, pp. 14–19. (In Tapper, 1978, *op. cit.*)

Feldman, M. and Feldman, H. (1973) The low-income liberated woman. *Human ecology forum* **4**: 13–16. (In Fransella, 1977, *op. cit.*)

Flowers, J., Whitley, J. and Cooper, C. (1978) *Assertion training: a general overview*. In Whitley, J. and Flowers, J. (eds), *Approaches to assertion training*. Monterey, CA: Brooks-Cole.

Forester, T.D. (1977) A description and evaluation of a life planning training program based on the self-empowerment construct: an explanatory study. *Dissertation abstracts international* **38**: (10–A) 6010.

Fransella, F. and Frost, K. (1977) *On being a woman – a review of research on how women see themselves*. Tavistock Women's Studies.

Freedman, M.J. (1968) Homosexuality among women and psychological adjustment. *Ladder* **12**: 2–3 (In Rosen, D. 1974, *op. cit.*)

French, J. and Adams, L. (1986) From analysis to synthesis: theories of health education. *Health education j.* **45** (2): 71–73.

Freud, S. (1933) *New introductory lectures on psychoanalysis*. New York: Norton.

Freymann, J.G. (1977) *The American health care system: its genesis and trajectory*. Huntington, NY: Robert E. Kreiger Pub. Co. (In Choi, 1985, *op. cit.*)

Furnham, A. (1979) Assertiveness in three cultures: multi-dimensionality and cultural differences. *J. of clinical psychology* **35** (3): 522–527.

Galassi, J.P. (1973) Assertive training in groups using video feedback. *Final progress report of National Institute of Mental Health small research grant MH22392–01*. (In Galassi and Galassi, 1978, *op. cit.*)

Galassi, M.D. and Galassi, J.P. (1978) Assertion: a critical review. *Psychotherapy: theory, research and practice* **15** (1): 16–29.

Gambarro, A. and Rabin S. (1969) Diastolic blood pressure response following direct and displaced aggression after anger arousal, in high and low guilt subjects. *J. of personality and social psychology* **12**: 87–94.

Gambrill, E. and Richey, C. (1975) An assertion inventory for use in assessment and research. *Behaviour therapy* **6**: 550–561.

Garrison, S. and O'Jenkins, J. (1986) Differing perceptions of black assertiveness as a function of race. *J. of multicultural counselling and development* **October**: 157–166.

Giesen, C. (1988) Becoming and remaining assertive: a longitudinal study. *Psychological reports* **63**: 595–605.

Gilchrist, L.D. and Schinke, S.P. (1983) Coping with contraception: cognitive and behavioural methods with adolescents. *Cognitive therapy research* **7**: 379–388.

Gildea. (1949) Special features of the personality which are common to certain psychosomatic disorders. *Psychosomatic medicine* **11**: 273–281. (In Brooks, 1980, *op. cit.*)

Halas, M. (1979) Sexism in women's medical care. *Frontiers* **4**: 11–15. (In Lindemann, 1984, *op. cit.*)

Hattem, J.V. (1964) Precipitating role of discordant interpersonal relationships in suicidal behaviour. *Dissertation abstracts international* **25**: 1335–6.

Haussmann, M. and Halseth, J. (1983) Re-examining women's roles: a feminist group approach to decreasing depression in women. *Social work with groups* **6** (3–4): 105–115.

Haynes, R.B., Taylor, R.W. and Sackett, D.L. (eds) (1979) *Compliance in health care*. Baltimore, M.D.: Johns Hopkins Univ. Press. (In Rabin *et al.*, 1986, *op. cit.*)

Heimberg, H., Montgomery, D., Madsen, C. and Heimberg, J. (1977) Assertion training: a review of the literature. *Behaviour therapy* **8**: 953–971.

Heiser, P. and Gannon, L. (1984) The relationship of sex-role stereotypy to anger expression and the report of psychosomatic symptoms. *Sex roles* **10** (7–8): 601–611.

Hirsche, S., Von Rosenberg, R., Phelan, C.S. and Dudley, H. (1978) The effectiveness of assertiveness training with alcoholics. *J. of studies on alcohol* **39** (1): 89–97.

Holandsworth, J.G. and Wall, K.E. (1977) Sex differences in assertive behaviour: an empirical investigation. *J. of counselling psychology* **24**: 217–222.

Holland, J., Ramazanoglu, C.R. and Scott, J.S. (1990) Young women and sexuality and the limitations of AIDS. *Gender and education.* (In press.) (Reported in *The Sunday Correspondent* 21 January 1990.)

Hopkins, J.M. (1969) The lesbian personality. *British j. of psychiatry* **115**: 1433–1436.

Hopson, B. and Scally, M. (1979) *Lifeskills teaching programmes.* Leeds University.

Hopson, B. and Scally, M. (1981) *Lifeskills teaching.* McGraw-Hill Book Co. (UK) Ltd.

Hynes, M.M. (1989) A school-based smoking prevention programme for adolescent girls in New York City. *Public health reports* **104** (1): 83–87.

Jakubowski, P. (1973) Facilitating the growth of women through assertiveness training. *Counselling psychologist.* **4**: 75–86.

Judge, J. (1985) Locus of control, self-empowerment and health education. Unpub. dissertation, HEA library.

Kagan, J. and Moss, H. (1962) *Birth to maturity: a study in psychological development.* New York: John Wiley & Sons.

Kann, L.K. (1987) Effects of computer-assisted instruction on selected interaction skills related to responsible sexuality. *J. of school health* **57** (7): 282–287.

Kaplan, H. (1973) Self-derogation and social position: interaction effects of sex, race, education and age. *Social psychology* **8**: 92–99. (In Fransella, 1977, *op. cit.*)

Keith, R.A. (1984) Functional assessment measures in medical rehabilitation: current status. *Archives of physical and medical rehabilitation* **65**: 74–78. (In Nosek, 1987, *op. cit.*)

Kelley, H., Berscheid, E., Christensen, L. and Harvey, J. (1983) *Close relationships.* New York: Freeman Press.

Kincaid, M. (1978) Assertiveness training from the participants' perspective. *Professional psychology* **9** (1): 153–160.

Kolbe, L., Iverson, D., Kreuter, M., Hochbaum, G. and Christensen, G. (1981) Propositions for an alternative and complementary health paradigm. *Health education* **May/June**: 24–30.

Lanesee, R.R., Bands, F.R. and Keller, M.D. (1972) Smoking behaviour in a teenage population: a multi-variate conceptual approach. *American J. of public health* **62**. (In Del Greco, 1980, *op. cit.*)

Lazarus, A. (1972) *Behaviour therapy and beyond.* (2nd edn) New York: McGraw-Hill.

Lehne, G.K. (1974) Homophobia among men. In David, D.S. and Brannon, R. (eds) *The forty-nine per cent majority – the male sex role*, p.66. (1976) Addison-Wesley Pub. Co.

Lindemann, C. (1984) Women's health/sexuality: the case of menopause. *J. of social work and human sexuality* **2** (1): 101–112.

Lindenfield, G. (1986) *Assert yourself – self help course.* Wellingborough: Thorsons.

Lineberger, M. and Calhoun, K. (1983) Assertive behaviour in black and white American undergraduates. *J. of psychology* **113**: 139–148.

Lirette, N.M. (1979) Psychosocial health, assertive behaviour and attitudes towards women's roles. PhD. thesis, Univ. of Calif.

Lomont, J.F., Gilner, F.H., Spector, N.J. and Skinner, K.K. (1969) Group assertion training and group insight therapies. *Psychological reports* **25**: 463–470.

Loney, J. (1972) Background factors, sexual experience and attitudes towards treatment in two 'normal' homosexual samples. *J. of consulting and clinical psychology* **38**: 57–65. (In Rosen, 1974, *op. cit.*)

Loo, C. (1982) Chinatown's wellness: an enclave of problems. *J. of the Asian American psychological association* **7** (1): 13–18.

Lowenstein, L.F. (1977) Who is the bully? *Home and school* **11**: 3–4.

MacDonald, M.L. (1975) Teaching assertion: a paradigm for therapeutic intervention. *Psychotherapy: theory, research and practice* **12**: 60–67.

Maslow, A. (1970) *Motivation and personality*. New York: Harper and Row.

McMillan, M.M. (1975) Relative efficacy of assertive training and self-control in a weight control program. Arizona Univ. *Dissertation abstracts international* 4265–A.

Minski, L. and Desai, M.M. (1955) Aspects of personality in peptic ulcer patients. *British J. of medical psychology* **28**: 113–134. (In Brooks, 1980, *op. cit.*)

Moore, D. (1979) *Battered women*. Beverley Hills, London: Sage.

Morford, M.L. and Barclay, L.K. (1984) Counselling the pregnant woman: implications for birth outcomes. *Personnel and guidance J.* **62** (10): 619–623.

Nosek, M.A., Parker, R.M. and Larsen, S. (1987) Psychosocial independence and functional abilities: their relationship in adults with severe musculoskeletal impairments. *Archives of physical and medical rehabilitation* **68** (12): 840–845.

Olzak, P. and Goldman, J. (1981) Relationship between self-actualisation and assertiveness in males and females. *Psychological reports* **48** (3): 931–937.

Pattenson, L. (1981) Homosexuality and health. Unpub. dissertation, Leeds Poly.

Percell, L. and Berwick, P. (1974) The effects of assertive training on self-concept and anxiety. *Archives of general psychiatry* **31**: 502–504.

Petrie, K. and Rotherham, M. (1982) Insulators against stress: self-esteem and assertiveness. *Psychological reports* **50**: 963–966.

Petrucco, O. and Harris, R. (1982) A psychology and demographic study of women patients with nonorganic pelvic pain. Paper presented at 8th New Zealand Congress, Auckland, New Zealand. In Broome and Wallace (1984) *Psychology and gynaecological problems*. London: Tavistock Publications.

Phelps, S. and Austin, N. (1987) *Assertive women: a new look*. San Luis Obispo, CA: Impact.

Pill, R. and Stott, N. (1985) Choice or chance: further evidence on ideas of illness and responsibility for health. *Social science and medicine* **20** (10): 981–999.

Price, J.L. and Collins, J.R. (1973) Smoking among baccalaureate nursing students. *Nursing research* **22**. (In Del Greco, 1980, *op. cit.*)

Rabin, C. and Amir, S. (1984) Prediction of compliance and control in juvenile diabetes through cognitive and assertive behaviour determinants. Unpub. manuscript, Tel Aviv Univ. (In Rabin *et al.*, 1986, *op. cit.*)

Rabin, C., Amir, S., Nardi, R. and Ovadia, B. (1986) Compliance and control issues in group training for diabetics. *Health and social work* **11** (2): 141–151.

Rainwater, M. *et al.* (1982) Teaching self-management skills to increase diet compliance in diabetics. In Stuart, R.B. (ed.), *Adherence, compliance and generalisation in behavioural medicine*. New York: Brunner/Mazel.

Rakusen, G. (1989) *The menopause – a guide for women of all ages*. Health Education Authority/National Extension College.

Rakusen, G. and Phillips, A. (1990) *Our bodies, ourselves: a health handbook for and by women*. London: Penguin.

Rathus, S. (1972) An experimental investigation of assertive training in a group setting. *J. of behaviour therapy and experimental psychiatry* **3**: 81–86.

Rathus, S. (1973) A 30-item schedule for assessing assertive behaviour. *Behaviour therapy* **4**: 389–406.

Rathus, S. (1975) Principles and practice of assertion training: an eclectic overview. *The counseling psychologist* **5** (4): 9–21.

Ray, J.J. and Lovejoy, F.H. (1984) The great androgyny myth: sex roles and mental health in the community at large. *J. of social psychology* **124** (2): 237–246.

Reagan, P. (1981) Introducing women's self-help in the curriculum. *Health education* **May/June**: 37–39.

Rich, A.R. and Schroeder, H.E. (1976) Research issues in assertiveness training **83**: 1081–1108.

Roberts, C.J., Elfriede, F. and Lillick, L.C. (1970) Association of psycho-social factors to the smoking practices of high school students. *Chronic disease* **17** (*supplement*). (In Del Greco, 1980, *op. cit.*)

Rogers, C. (1979) A film review of 'Five women, five births: a film about choices'. *Women and health* **4**: 196–198. (In Lindemann, 1984, *op. cit.*)

Rogers, C.R. (1951) *Client centred therapy.* Boston, MA: Houghton-Mifflin. (In Rathus, 1975, *op. cit.*)

Rogers, C.R. (1963) The concept of the fully functioning person. *Psychotherapy: theory, research and practice* **1**: 17–26 (In Rathus, 1975, *op. cit.*)

Rohrbach, L.A., Graham, J.W., Hansen, W.B., Flay, B.R. and Johnson, C.A. (1987) Evaluation of resistance skills using multi-trait – multi-method role play skill assessments. *Health education research theory and practice* **2** (4): 401–407.

Rosen, D. (1974) *Lesbianism – a study of female homosexuality.* IL: C.C. Thomas.

Rosenkrantz, P., Vogel, S., Bee, Broverman, I. and Broverman, D. (1968) Sex role stereotypes and self-concept in college students. *J. of consulting and clinical psychology* **32**: 287–295.

Rosenstock, I.M., Strecher, V.J. and Becker, M.H. (1988) Social learning theory and the health belief model. *Health education quarterly* **Summer 1988**: 175–183.

Rotter, J. (1966) Generalized expectancies for internal versus external control of reinforcement. *Psychological monographs* **80** (1): p. 609.

Saghir, M. and Robins, E. (1971) Male and female homosexuality: natural history. *Comprehensive psychiatry* **12**: 503–510.

Salber, E.J., Reed, R.B., Harrison, S.V. and Green, J.H. (1963) Smoking behaviour, recreational activities and attitudes towards smoking among Newton secondary school children. *Pediatrics* **32**. (In Del Greco, 1980, *op. cit.*)

Salber, E.J., Welsh, B. and Taylor, S.V. (1971) Reasons for smoking given by secondary school children. *J. of health and human behaviour* **4**. (In Del Greco, 1980, *op. cit.*)

Salter, A. (1949) *Conditional reflex therapy*. New York: Creative Age. (In Furnham, 1979, *op. cit.*)

Sanchez, V.S. and Lewinsohn, P. (1979) Assertive behaviour and depression. *J. of consulting and clinical psychology* **48** (1): 119–120.

Sanchez, V., Lewinsohn, P. and Larson, D. (1980) Assertiveness training and depression. *J. of clinical psychology* **36** (2): 526–529.

Schofield, M. (1965) *Sociological aspects of homosexuality*. Longmans, Green and Co.

Schnieder, F.W. and Vanmastrigi, L.A. (1974) Adolescent-preadolescent differences in beliefs and attitudes about cigarette smoking. *J. of psychology* **87**. (In Del Greco, 1980, *op. cit.*)

Sears, R.R. (1961) Relation of early socialisation experiences to aggression in middle childhood. *J. of abnormal and social psychology* **64**: 466–492.

Sedgewick, A., Paul, B., Plooj, D. and Davies, M. (1989) Follow-up of stress management courses. *Medical journal of Australia* **150** (9): 485–9.

Serber, M. (1972) Teaching the non-verbal components of assertion training. *J. of behaviour therapy and experimental psychiatry* **3**: 179–183.

Shafer, R.B. (1988) Equity, inequity and self-esteem – a reassessment. *Psychological reports* **63** (2): 637–638.

Siegelman, M. (1972) Adjustment of homosexual and heterosexual women. *British J. of psychiatry* **120**: 477–481. (In Rosen, 1974, *op. cit.*)

Sifneos, P.E., (1970) The doctor-patient relationship in manipulative suicide, a common psychosomatic disease. *Pschotherapy and psychosomatics* **18**: 40–46. (In Tapper, 1978, *op. cit.*)

Soto, E. and Shaver, P. (1982) Sex role traditionalism, assertiveness and symptoms of Puerto Rican women living in the United States. *Hispanic J. of behavioural sciences* **4** (1): 1–19.

Spence, J.T., Helmreich, R. and Stapp, J. (1974) The personal attribute questionnaire: a measure of sex role stereotypes and masculinity – femininity. *JSAS catalogue of selected documents in psychology* **4**: 127.

Strecher, V.J., DeVellis, B.E., Becker, M.H. and Rosenstock, I.M. (1986) The role of self-efficacy in achieving health behaviour change. *Health education quarterly* **Spring**: 73–92.

Stuart, R.B. (ed.) (1982) *Adherence, compliance and generalisation in behavioural medicine*. New York: Brunner/Mazel. (In Rabin *et al.*, 1986, *op. cit.*)

Tanck, R.Q. and Robbins, P. (1979) Assertiveness, locus of control and coping behaviours used to diminish tension. *J. of personality assessment*. **43**: 396–400.

Tapper, B.J. (1978) Assertion training in suicidal and depressed clients. In *Approaches to assertion training*. Whiteley, J.M. and Flowers, J.V. (eds) Brooks/Cole Series in *Counselling psychology*, Monterey.

Thompson, N., McCaudless, B. and Strickland, B. (1971) Personal adjustment of male and female homosexuals and heterosexuals. *J. of abnormal psychology* **78**: 237–240. (In Rosen, 1974, *op. cit.*)

Tones, B.K. (1986) Health education and the ideology of health promotion: a review of alternative approaches. *Health education research theory and practice* **1** (1): 3–12.

Troutt, B.V. (1980) Independence and ego identity reflected in minority students utilisation of support services in academic special program. *Dissertation abstracts international* **41** (5–A): 2029. (In Nosek, 1987, *op. cit.*)

Verbrugge, L. (1983) Multiple roles and physical health of women and men. *J. of health and social behaviour* **24**: 16–30.

Wark, M.A. (1980) Sex-role stereotyping and health. Unpub. dissertation, Leeds Poly.

WEA (Workers Educational Association) (1988) *Health education for women: a report and evaluation of work in the WEA north western district.* London: Amazon Press.

Weinberg, G. and Williams. (1974) *Male homosexuals.* New York, London: Oxford University Press.

Weissman, M. and Klerman, G. (1977) Sex-differences and the epidemiology of depression. *Archives of general psychiatry* **34**: 98–111.

Wesson, N. (1988) *The assertive pregnancy – a guide to the alternatives in childbirth.* Wellingborough: Grapevine.

Whitehead, C. (1990) *Assertiveness and women's health education.* Health Education Authority publication.

Williams, J. (1987) *Psychology of women.* (3rd edn). London: Norton & Co.

Williams, J. and Stout, J. (1985) The effect of high and low assertiveness on locus of control and health problems. *J. of psychology* **119** (2): 169–173.

Wolf, J. and Fodor, I. (1975) A cognitive behavioural approach to modifying assertive behaviour in women. *Counselling psychologist* **5**: 45–52.

Wolpe, J. (1958) *Psychotherapy by reciprocal inhibition.* Stanford Univ. Press. (In Furnham, 1979, *op. cit.*)

Wolpe, J. (1969) *The practice of behavior therapy.* New York: Pergamon.

WHO (World Health Organisation) (1985) *Targets for health for all.* Copenhagen.

Zagona, S.V. and Zurcher, L.A. (1965) An analysis of some psychosocial variables associated with smoking behaviour in a college sample. *Psychological reports* **17**. (In Del Greco, 1980, *op. cit.*)